Get fit
with the
Green Goddess

Diana Moran

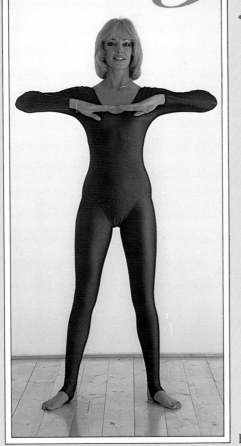

BRITISH BROADCASTING CORPORATION

Photographs by Bob Komar
Cover photographs and photographs on pages 32 and 33
© BBC by Les Wilson, Topical Production Centre, Lime Grove

Published by the British Broadcasting Corporation
35 Marylebone High Street, London W1M 4AA

ISBN 0 563 20213 0

First published 1983
© Diana Moran Limited, 1983

Set in 11/13 Cheltenham Light by Garland Graphics Limited, Bristol
Printed and bound in Great Britain by Chorley and Pickersgill Limited, Leeds

A BBC LP and cassette of *Get Fit with the Green Goddess*
are available from record shops.

Contents

Introduction 7

'The Great Stretch' 16–17

PART 1: THE HEAD, NECK AND SHOULDERS

Head Roll 18

Neck 19

Neck and Shoulders 20–21

Shoulders and Upper Arms 22–23

PART 2: THE BACK AND CHEST

Back 24

Bottom and Back 25

Boobs and Under Arms 26

Chest and Upper Arms 27

Chest and Under Arms 28–29

PART 3: THE WAIST AND TUMMY

Waist 30–31

'On Location' 32–33

Waist and Back 34–35

Tummy 36–37

Tummy and Thighs 38–39

Tummy and Hips 40–41

Middle 42–43

Hips 44–45

PART 4: THE LEGS AND BOTTOM

Bottom and Thighs 46–47

Bottom and Legs 48–49

Thighs 50–51

Knees 52

Thighs and Bottom 53

Calves 54

Spine 55

Ankles 56

Feet 57

'Pass Out' 58

PART 5: VARIATIONS

Tummy and Thighs 59

Tummy and Legs 60

General Stretch 61

General Mobility 62–63

'My Personal Pick-Me-Up' 64

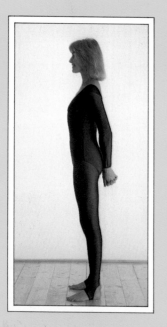

These exercises should not be attempted if you are in poor health, suffer from a bad back or are pregnant. If in doubt, please check with your doctor before starting any programme of exercise.

It is *essential* to warm up the entire body ('The Great Stretch', page 16) at the start of each session.

Begin gently and gradually, build up daily, listen to your body and don't overstrain. The movements will become easier with practice as the body gains flexibility.

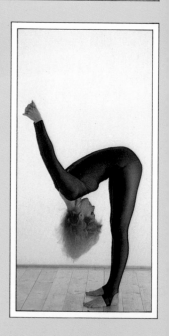

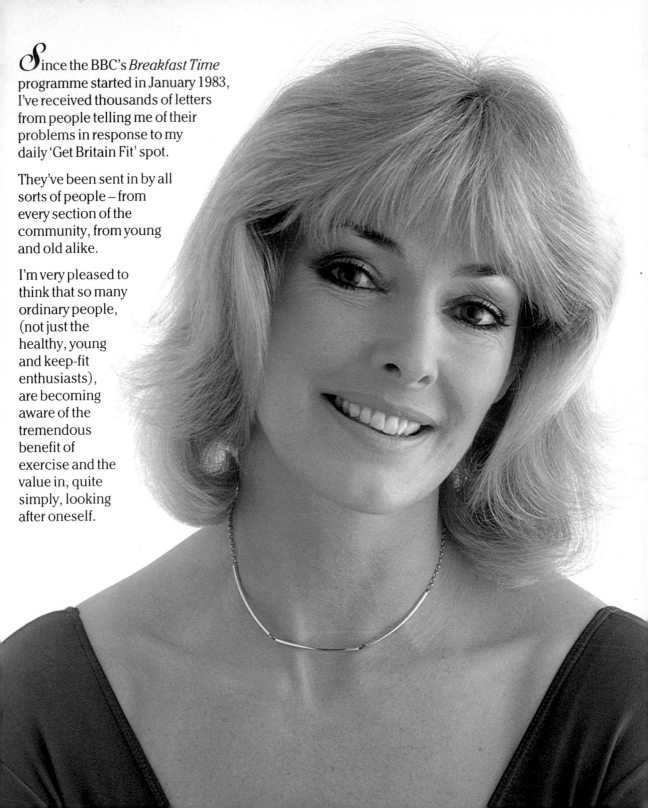

$\mathcal{S}$ince the BBC's *Breakfast Time* programme started in January 1983, I've received thousands of letters from people telling me of their problems in response to my daily 'Get Britain Fit' spot.

They've been sent in by all sorts of people – from every section of the community, from young and old alike.

I'm very pleased to think that so many ordinary people, (not just the healthy, young and keep-fit enthusiasts), are becoming aware of the tremendous benefit of exercise and the value in, quite simply, looking after oneself.

*A*ll too often, we take what Nature has given us for granted – we don't appreciate what we have until it's too late.

It's crazy isn't it? We buy a car and prize it. We clean it, study it, spend time and money on it and keep it up to scratch. We listen to it – take advice about it – and regularly service it. We fuel and water it correctly, and for our pains we expect it to respond by running efficiently. And it pleases us and we commend ourselves when it does.

So why don't we cosset ourselves and our bodies in the same way? It's a fine piece of construction we've each of us been given free, at our birth. It would, surely, make very good sense. But no, we're too busy, too lazy, or are we just too ignorant? Perhaps that's what it is. We're not aware of the facts, we haven't thought that we *need* to do something about it – no, we've just taken it all for granted. But at some time or other in our lives we're forced to stop and think – because, just like that car, sometimes *we* break down and come to a standstill – or just little bits of us do. Our previously efficient bodies won't run well until some adjustments are made.

I am a great one for thinking that Nature has its own way in the end. It stops us in our tracks every now and again most inconveniently, and particularly when we've been pushing our engine just a little *too* hard; we've failed to pay attention to the fine tuning of our bodies or perhaps we have neglected to fuel it properly. Maybe we've substituted the wrong type of food because it was more convenient. Unlike a car, our fuel has to provide energy *and* do body repair work all at the same time. But like a car we need regular fuel to give us the energy to keep us moving. Our energy is in the form of food containing calories. What exactly is a calorie? It is a measurement of the energy contained in all the food we eat *and* drink. The car's fuel tank will just simply overflow when full but we *can* overfill ourselves, and, when we do, the excess gets stored around our body in the form of fat. So let's think for a moment about what we eat.

Exercise alone will not slim – it will, however, firm and trim and tone the body. The only way to lose weight effectively is to eat less. Think of a pair of

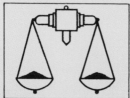

old-fashioned scales, and I'll explain the calorie balance. On one side we have the food we eat which contains 'calories'. (Remember a calorie is a measure of the energy in that food). On the other side we have the amount of energy our body requires daily. This, of course, is going to vary enormously from person to person, depending upon their age, sex, work, health and metabolism. We each have to learn for ourselves how to keep the scales balanced. The number of calories we put into our body through our daily food must correspond to the calories our bodies use up each day. If not, the excess calories get stored up around our bodies in the form of fat. When we reduce our calorie intake the extra energy required by the body will be taken from those 'fat stores' (thighs, bottom, tums etc.) and the result is that we lose weight. So, we must educate and look after ourselves more, if we want to keep our bodies running well. We may not extend our lives any longer by doing so, but we will certainly add *more* life and efficiency to the years that we do have.

A spell in hospital twelve years ago made me realise all this – which is just old-fashioned common sense. I was fortunate enough to have had a normal healthy childhood, and an active and sporty adolescence. I had a young athletic body – highly tuned and efficient. I married when I was still in my teens, and immediately began producing my family with the usual amount of fuss and bother. I didn't think *too* much about my physical well-being – 'Nature will look after its own', and fortunately it more or less did! Then like most mothers, I became *completely* absorbed in bringing up my brood and most of the time I forgot about myself. Indeed, there wasn't much alternative for me to do anything else, I was inexperienced, unsure and without any help or my own mother's invaluable advice. My mother died when I was in my mid-teens, and oh, how I *did* envy all my girlfriends the support of their mothers, the one thing in my life that has caused me to feel the stinging pains of jealousy. Yet *another* example of taking things, or people, for granted until they're not there any more. So, I just got on with the job – tiring and exhausting as it was – it totally fulfilled all my strong maternal instincts. Gardening, which I love, was all that helped me to stay reasonably fit.

Suddenly, and unexpectedly, I found myself in hospital. The boys were cared for by friends and for a few weeks I was on my own, with time to concentrate on just me and getting my strength back after a throat operation. And for the very first time I realised that good health was of premier importance. Not only for oneself but for all one's dependants. It colours all that we can do, and I decided there and then to take better care of myself for the sake of all the family. I saw that I was out of tune and my body needed toning, for without being aware of it I had let myself go since the children were born, and now was the time to do something about it. I had always wanted to get back to some form of sport but knew that organised activities could not be fitted into my busy schedule – for by then I was modelling part-time, the work growing enormously with my availability since the boys were now, of course, at school. And that's where and how Keep Fit came into my life. I read books, particularly on Yoga, which attracted me, and the classic Keep Fit routines. But full Yoga positions weren't possible for me because I had lost the necessary flexibility. I was too old to start Aerobics, being a little concerned at the exhaustive element of these movements for other than the young. I discovered from many sources a variety of exercise programmes and, over the next few years experimented on myself, reaping the benefits. I combined these exercises with a study of diet and eating habits. This was precipitated by a sudden appendix operation, and while in hospital I learnt a great deal about cellulose, roughage and the benefits of a high fibre diet.

Soon I felt better – in fact I positively glowed, and coped with more work, more family responsibilities and many charitable and welfare commitments. People began to comment upon my healthy looks, my achievements and my capacity for hard work – upon which I seemed to thrive.

A few years later I was asked to take regular keep fit classes at a large holiday camp and received tuition to help me to do so. I was very apprehensive as I stood in front of my first large class of several hundred ordinary people, men, women, and children, all holidaymakers rather than keep fit enthusiasts. I was delighted by their response to me and my simple keep fit programme, and from then on I have not looked back.

A producer at HTV, my local television station, who knew I worked as a keep fit instructor asked me to do a spot for a magazine programme he was planning. I did. It was successful and resulted in my own spot for three years in the network series *Here Today*. At the same time my work as a fashion and photographic model disciplined me to keep my figure at the required size twelve. Eventually I began to pass on my findings regarding exercising, along with my extensive knowledge of the modelling business as a whole, to young aspirants, whom I trained, whilst attending modelling schools.

*K*eep fit has become an important way of life for me and, over the past months, a most enjoyable job of work as well. My methods are based on a mixture of Yoga, Isometrics, and classic exercises and are drawn from extensive research and a close look at all forms of keeping oneself fit. My approach, which is basic, and beneficial, seems to be an inspiration for Mr and Mrs Average, Granny, Grandpa, and the kids too, and I am thrilled to be able to pass on my findings to millions of viewers via the medium of BBC *Breakfast*

Time with a programme of exercise which will help us *all* make the most of ourselves. Basically, we must recondition our bodies, especially in adult life. We must develop new habits that are to become a way of life. We must learn to watch what we eat and drink, and take some sort of exercise. All too often, as adults, we overeat and under-exercise. We must also 'get comfortable' with ourselves – aim for a personal goal, *but* a realistic one. No point in trying to 'think thin' when, in fact, your basic shape and bone structure is heavy or large. That would only lead to constant frustration and unhappiness. No, far better to settle for a compromise, and to *reach* your target. A weight and size at which you feel, look, and are, healthy and happy. *Then* stick to it!

MEN

Height without shoes ft in	Small frame st lb st lb	Medium frame st lb st lb	Large frame st lb st lb
5 1	8 0- 8 8	8 6- 9 3	9 0-10 1
5 2	8 3- 8 12	8 9- 9 7	9 3-10 4
5 3	8 6- 9 0	8 12- 9 10	9 6-10 8
5 4	8 9- 9 3	9 1- 9 13	9 9-10 12
5 5	8 12- 9 7	9 4-10 3	9 12-11 2
5 6	9 2- 9 11	9 8-10 7	10 2-11 7
5 7	9 6-10 1	9 12-10 12	10 7-11 12
5 8	9 10-10 5	10 2-11 2	10 11-12 2
5 9	10 0-10 10	10 6-11 6	11 1-12 6
5 10	10 4-11 0	10 10-11 11	11 5-12 11
5 11	10 8-11 4	11 0-12 2	11 10-13 2
6 0	10 12-11 8	11 4-12 7	12 0-13 7
6 1	11 2-11 13	11 8-12 12	12 5-13 12
6 2	11 6-12 3	11 13-13 3	12 10-14 3
6 3	11 10-12 7	12 4-13 8	13 0-14 8

WOMEN

Height without shoes ft in	Small frame st lb st lb	Medium frame st lb st lb	Large frame st lb st lb
4 8	6 8- 7 0	6 12- 7 9	7 6- 8 7
4 9	6 10- 7 3	7 0- 7 12	7 8- 8 10
4 10	6 12- 7 6	7 3- 8 1	7 11- 8 13
4 11	7 1- 7 9	7 6- 8 4	8 0- 9 2
5 0	7 4- 7 12	7 9- 8 7	8 3- 9 5
5 1	7 7- 8 1	7 12- 8 10	8 6- 9 8
5 2	7 10- 8 4	8 1- 9 0	8 9- 9 12
5 3	7 13- 8 7	8 4- 9 4	8 13-10 2
5 4	8 2- 8 11	8 8- 9 9	9 3-10 6
5 5	8 6- 9 1	8 12- 9 13	9 7-10 10
5 6	8 10- 9 5	9 2-10 3	9 11-11 0
5 7	9 0- 9 9	9 6-10 7	10 1-11 4
5 8	9 4-10 0	9 10-10 11	10 5-11 9
5 9	9 8-10 4	10 0-11 1	10 9-12 0
5 10	9 12-10 8	10 4-11 5	10 13-12 5

*L*et's just have a brief word about our diets remembering that exercise alone doesn't make us lose weight. Exercising will certainly trim and tone up our bodies making us feel well, and can help reshape and improve those bulges and flab. But, if your clothes feel tight and you can't squeeze into those trousers, then it's time you did the 'pinch test'! With your thumb and forefinger pinch yourself: under the arm, just above your bra, around the hips, top of the thighs. What about that bot and your 'spare tyre'? More than an inch of flab? Then it's time to do something about it. Middle age spread *is* avoidable, an increase in years shouldn't be an excuse for extra inches. And it *isn't* inevitable for you to lose your figure after childbirth. The way to shape up is a combination of exercise and diet. So, learn to watch your diet and find out about the calorie content of the food you eat *and* drink.

Beware of oily, fatty foods high in calories. But do eat lots of fresh fruit and vegetables which are low in calories and full of vitamins. There's an added bonus too, your skin will improve – you'll have a clear glowing complexion and far fewer spots.

Bulky foods such as cereals and wholemeal breads are high in fibre content and will help avoid digestive problems and constipation.

Cut down on your calorie intake by watching the *fat* content whilst you're cooking your meals. Cut off visible fat from all meats. Throw away the frying pan, grill your meats, sausages and bacon instead. You'll be amazed at the amount of fat you can then throw away and avoid! When you're shopping, choose leaner cuts of meats or have chicken, offal, fish or eggs instead, they contain fewer calories. Substitute butter and margarine with a low fat spread, and if you've a sweet tooth why not use an artificial sweetener instead of sugar? And watch those sauces, gravies and salad creams. They're rich in calories and will soon bump up your calorie intake. Do remember that those little 'nibbles', crisps, nuts and cocktail biscuits may only be small, but, they're heavy in calories. And finally, don't forget that what you *drink* is important. Sweet fizzy drinks, beers, ciders, sweet wines and sherries must also be taken into consideration for your personal calorie intake, since they too have a high calorie content and *all too easily* can add on those extra unwanted inches!

Two extra little hints to help you 'fight the flab'. Try putting *your* food on a smaller plate than the rest of the family when you dish up. In that way you'll eat less without noticing! And do take care not to become your family's 'Dustbin' by eating up all those leftovers. Many, many Mums can't bear to see waste and ruin their figures by popping what the children leave, into their own mouths. That, and constant 'tasting' whilst cooking must be the two biggest traps to fall into. The calories in those ounces soon turn into pounds – 3,500 calories are equal to 1 lb of body fat – so for your own sake, avoid them!

Real health and beauty comes from within and is then radiated out. So forget the gadgets, the gimmicks and the creams, and learn self-discipline and determination. You'll be surprised and delighted with the results, if you persevere.

*S*ome people benefit from this combination of diet and exercise more quickly than others. Our metabolism (which is nature's mechanism for changing our food into energy) works at different rates in different people. These rates we are born with and cannot basically be altered, so this must be taken into consideration, since they vary a great deal from one individual to another. We have to know ourselves. And eventually we will lose weight, when we become fully aware of *all* of ourselves and our habits, which up until now we've taken for granted. We ladies benefit at any age by our bodies becoming trimmer and firmer as we lose flab and weight. We can improve our posture with this new long look at ourselves and, along with this, gain confidence as we make the *most* of ourselves. The men will discover new strength and stamina and generally feel more active and fit and all of us will sleep better. Older people will acquire suppleness and added mobility – keeping their bodies a little more active for longer.

You don't have to be 'super-fit' to start these exercises. Many of the mild gentle stretches require only a little effort and after a few weeks of practice you will gain more control and then you'll be able to do more, and will really reap the advantages of the extra energy and mobility you'll experience. So 'little and often' – even as little as three minutes to begin with. Just a good 'stretch' will help greatly.

So – get motivated – perhaps encourage the family at home or join or form a group where you can profit from the discipline of a class. But do try to practise daily and at any time. Some of us prefer the mornings which, for me, naturally starts with the 'stretch' – just like a cat waking up in the mornings – we can all take a tip from Nature!

Others prefer the evening, when they can collapse into a hot bath and bed afterwards. Many young mums I know find a quiet time during the day. They know they can be alone, undisturbed in the house, and can exercise conscientiously to the rhythm of music from records or the radio in the privacy of their own home. Build up to half an hour of exercises a day (or more if you can spare the time). Use the Top to Toe Keep Fit Programme and then spend any extra minutes on your own individual 'problem' areas. We've *all* got them! So take heart and be honest with yourself. *You* alone know which yours are – so *attack* them and you'll feel so proud and pleased when after only a few weeks you can see an improvement. But keep at it and don't slack back again! It gets easier as you go on and eventually becomes a habit and part of *your* daily personal routine.

Learn generally how to loosen up your entire body – you'll be amazed at how quickly it responds. You'll feel less stiff and become more supple. Your muscles will be less cramped and tense and the result is that you'll feel younger. I met a lady of seventy from the Keep Fit Association, whilst filming one of the programmes, who had exercised for many years. Her philosophy was 'if you don't use – you'll lose it'. I think that certainly applies to many parts of our bodies (and perhaps our minds?!). So wake up those lazy muscles and move those joints, you'll add more health and enjoyment to your life whatever your age.

Let's stretch and strengthen parts of your body you had forgotten existed. Parts that haven't been regularly or methodically exercised for years. And if you *do* experience aches, pains or discomfort, simply stop for a day or so. Listen to your own body – you're the best judge, be sensible, stop when you feel you've reached your body's limit. Start gently and after three or so days you'll be surprised how easy it becomes. But *do* try hard.

*H*owever, never overstretch and strain, particularly if you've been *foolish* enough not to warm up the entire body and muscles to begin with. I find it beneficial to have a hot bath after an intensive work out, as this keeps any (or most) of the aches and pains at bay!

Exercise with little food in the stomach – which is why I find early mornings so good – and don't exercise until an hour after you've eaten.

Through all the movements, stretches and exercises, breathe normally. Deep, easy breaths. Don't hold the breath or become tense.

If you pant whilst exerting yourself, that's good. Breathe more deeply – fill the lungs with air – (even more beneficial if you're out of doors). More life-giving oxygen will be absorbed into the blood. The heart will beat faster and the circulation will improve. The increased stamina of the heart and lungs will result in a generally healthier body.

But there's no point in over-exerting yourself. I'm trying to help to keep you fit, not *exhaust* you by using up all your energy. **If you are in doubt about your state of health and haven't exercised for years, consult your doctor before starting a programme of exercise. Particularly if you have a bad back, a heart condition, or high blood pressure and, of course, if you are pregnant, you mustn't attempt the exercises.**

*C*lothing needs to be kept to a minimum to give you ease of movement. Just underclothes or, better still, nothing if you're in the privacy of your own home. Wear leotards, tights, shorts, track suits, if you're keen, or just loosen collars, belts, and buttons, to take advantage of a few minutes' practice. Practise wherever you can find enough space to allow you to move easily and throw yourself around a bit: the lounge, the bedroom, the hallway – I find the landing in my house the best area!

*Bare feet are best.
*Shoes with heels must be taken off.
*Beware of socks and tights in case you slip.

Carpet or a mat can make exercising less uncomfortable, especially the floor exercises.

So there we are – now we're ready.

Let's begin by stretching . . . . . .

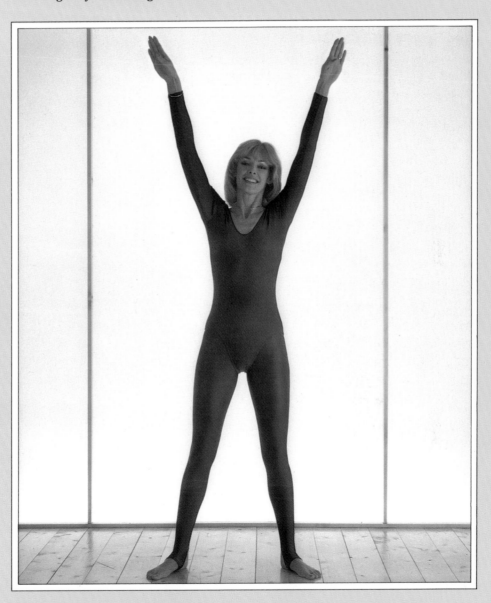

The Great Stretch

Let's begin by taking a tip from Nature – Wake up, stand up and STRETCH.

Just like a cat does after a long nap, extending and literally stretching the entire length of its body, flexing its muscles ready to spring into action.

It's my favourite exercise and always starts my day. It uses and warms up the whole body, makes the heart beat faster and gets the circulation moving. You will pant a bit and consequently breathe more deeply, filling your lungs with oxygen which soon gets absorbed into the blood stream – leaving you with a glowing sensation, a feeling of coming alive!

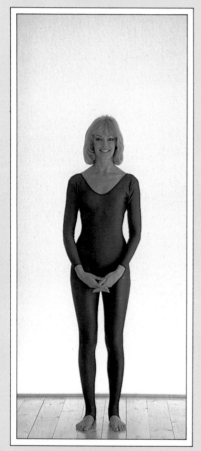

1 Stand with your feet apart, feel nice and easy

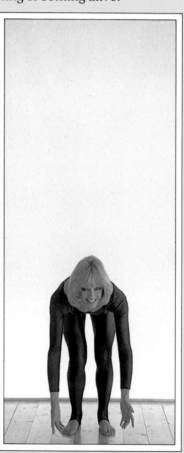

2 Bend the knees, take the arms down and back

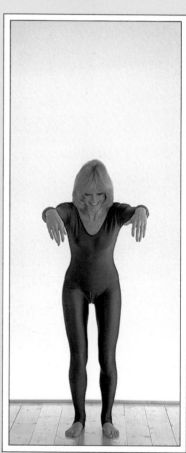

3 Swing arms up and forward, at the same time straightening the knees

And on days when you're short of time and can't do a complete exercise programme, at least *stretch*. You'll find that just three minutes stretching will make you tingle, increase your energy and leave you more alert to face the day.

With your body warmed up (an *essential* start to any exercise session) you're now ready to work out from top to toe. A complete Keep Fit programme which will take half to three-quarters of an hour and benefit the entire body. On busy days, however, always start with the 'great stretch' and then concentrate on your particular problem area. You know where it is! So work on it.

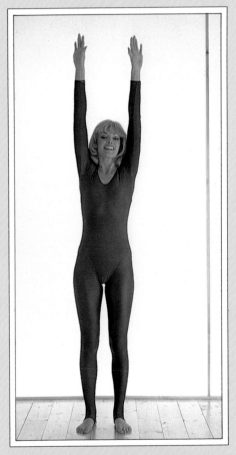

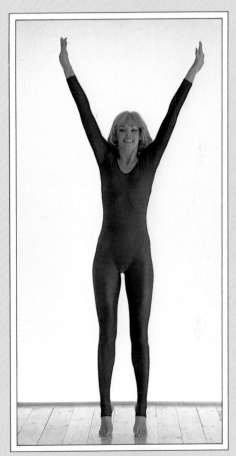

4 Swing arms up, high above head, lifting the rib cage. Stretch and pull up through the entire body

5 Expand chest, opening arms out a little and reaching up on tiptoe

Head Roll

Tensions quickly build up in the neck area and are often the cause of headaches, so release some of the stress by simply rolling your head, loosening the cramped neck muscles and relaxing.

- **Never do this exercise with the head leaning back.**

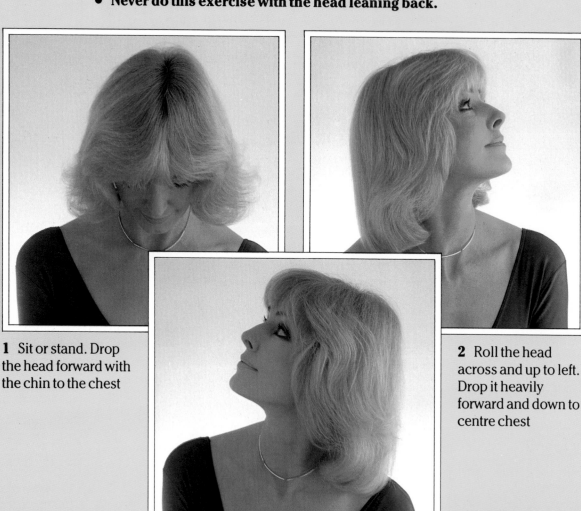

1 Sit or stand. Drop the head forward with the chin to the chest

2 Roll the head across and up to left. Drop it heavily forward and down to centre chest

3 Roll it on and up to right

- **REPEAT ABOUT 6 TIMES** •

Neck

While you're about it – why not do yourself a favour and prevent or improve that double chin!

This is a simple and effective exercise to tone up those lazy muscles which can soon sag if you constantly position your head down – especially those of you who work in an office all day.

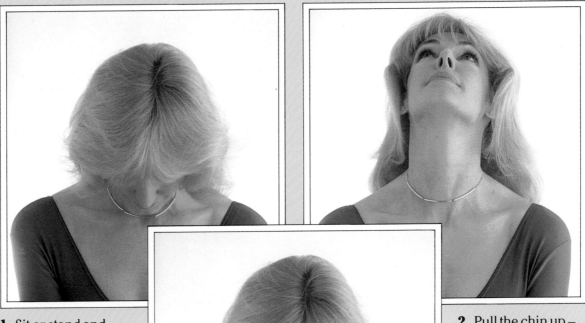

1 Sit or stand and drop head forward to the chest

2 Pull the chin up – mouth closed – and pull head firmly up and back – but don't jerk. Feel the taut muscles in the throat and chin. Hold for 5 seconds

3 Drop chin back to chest

• CONTINUE RHYTHMICALLY 6 TIMES •

Neck and Shoulders

We take the troubles of the world upon our shoulders.

Just watch small children timidly lift up their shoulders when they're worried or afraid. With words of kindness the shoulders drop down again and they come out of their shells.

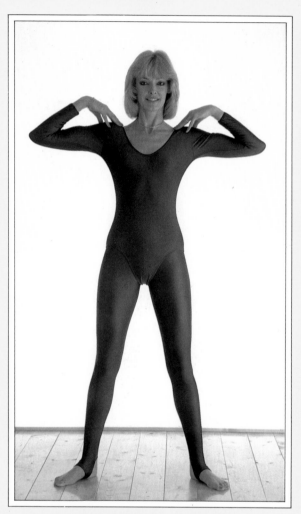

1 Sit or stand and place fingertips on top of shoulders

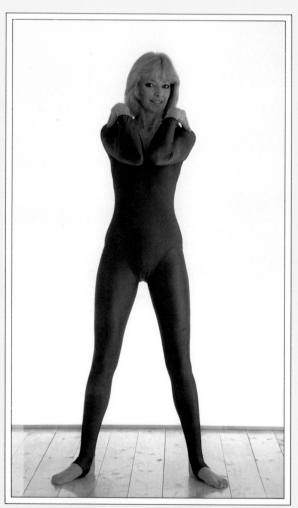

2 Bring elbows together in front of chest

As adults we often suffer from anxiety, but have learnt to cover-up the signs in order to disguise our inner feelings. Nevertheless the stresses and strains are still there which build up around the neck and shoulders in the form of tension. Here are some exercises to rid yourself of it.

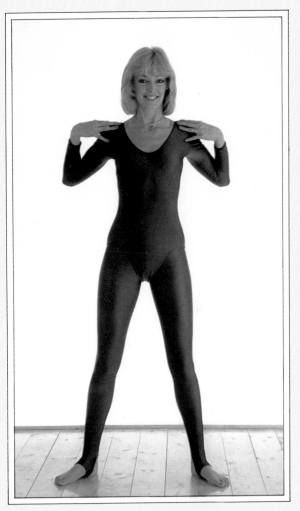

4 Circle elbows back, pulling shoulder blades together

Continue down, back, then forward, completing the circle

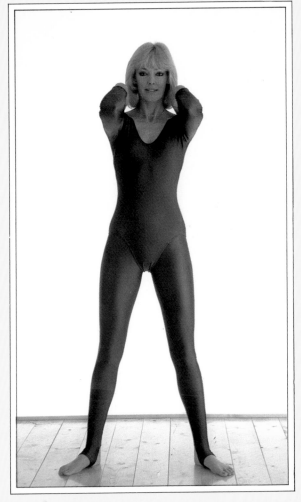

3 Circle elbows up and over, with the fingertips still in original position

Shoulders and Upper Arms

This useful exercise keeps the shoulders flexible, tones the upper arms plus expanding the chest.

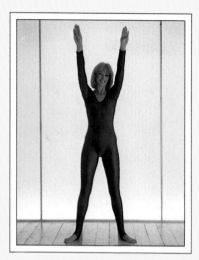

1 Stand with feet apart and raise arms in the air

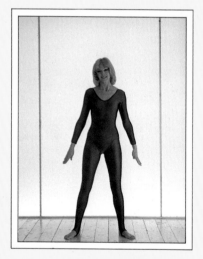

2 Drop arms forward and down and back

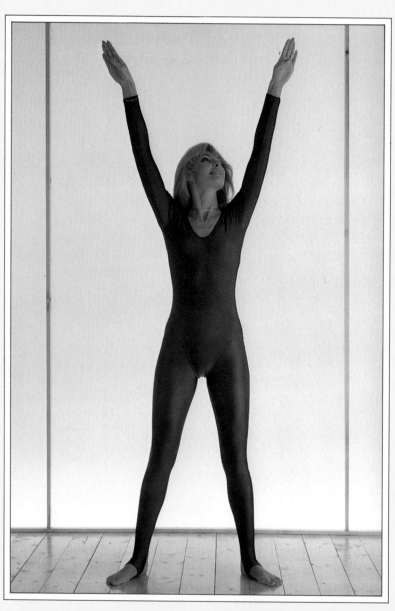

3 Gaining momentum, swing arms forward and up

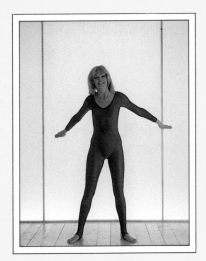

4 Continue swinging the arms back to complete the circle with big, strong movements

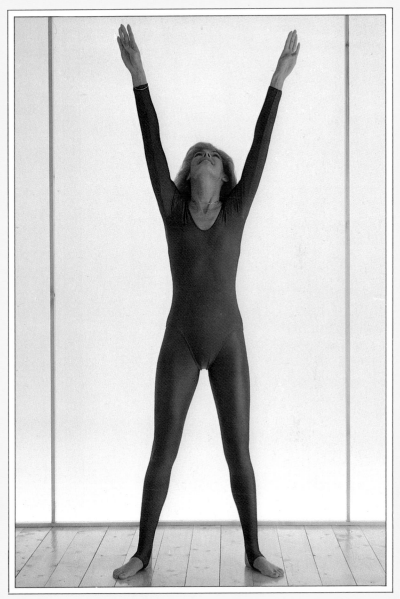

5 Arms up again with a good stretch

23

Back

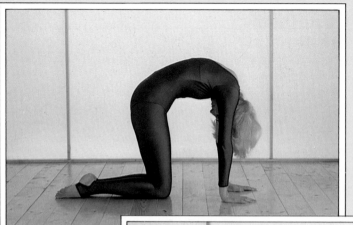

Many people suffer from back ache at some time or another in their lives. 'Bad Backs' cause the loss of many working days. A strong supple back can *prevent* strain and damage. So let's strengthen it with another lesson from Nature, and again that cat!

● **Remember if you have a bad back, to seek medical advice before attempting this and subsequent back exercises**.

1 Kneel down on all fours with your hands flat on the floor, shoulder width apart. Knees and feet a little apart. Drop head down to chest, pull up the tummy, clench the bottom and arch up the spine, without jerking, like a cat waking up. Hold for 3 seconds

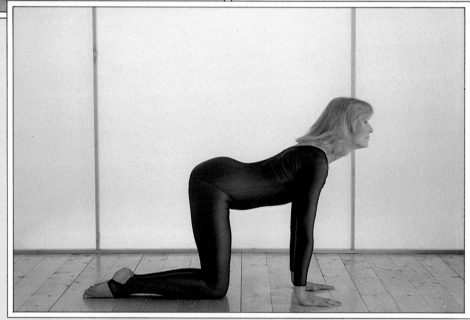

2 Raise the head and look up. At the same time curve down the spine, push the bottom up and out. Hollow the back as much as possible and hold for three seconds

● REPEAT 6 TIMES STRONGLY AND SMOOTHLY ●

This exercise can relieve menstrual pain and is particularly beneficial after child birth. It is safe to do after your post-natal check

Bottom and Back

This is a variation which will help strengthen the back as well as firming your bottom.

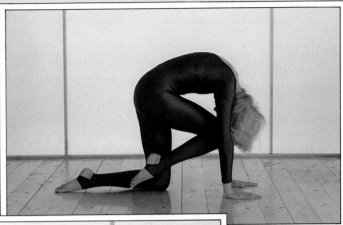

1 Start in the same position as before – on all fours. Drop the head down and at the same time bring forward the right knee to touch the head

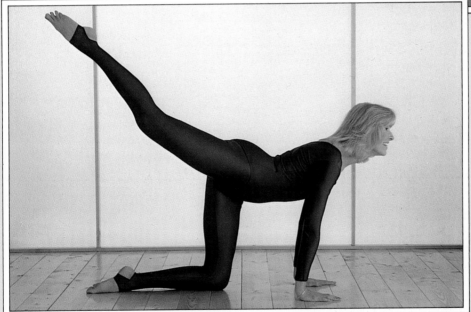

2 With a strong, smooth movement, lift head up and look out, hollowing the back. At the same time straighten and lift the right leg back and up high, and hold

● **REPEAT 6 TIMES WITH STRONG SMOOTH MOVEMENTS THEN REPEAT WITH LEFT KNEE** ●

Boobs and Under Arms

Women are rarely satisfied with the shape Nature has given them. Many would like to change shape – a little more here, or a little less there!

The bust, along with the hips, is one of these areas – but *unlike* the hips the bust size is not easily altered. You can however strengthen the pectoral muscles – those supporting the breasts and give the bust an uplift!

This is also good for chest expansion – therefore men can benefit too!

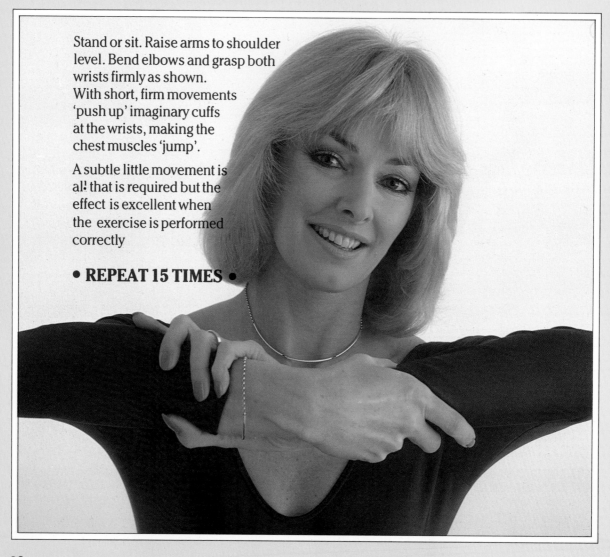

Stand or sit. Raise arms to shoulder level. Bend elbows and grasp both wrists firmly as shown. With short, firm movements 'push up' imaginary cuffs at the wrists, making the chest muscles 'jump'.

A subtle little movement is al! that is required but the effect is excellent when the exercise is performed correctly

● **REPEAT 15 TIMES** ●

Chest and Upper Arms

Arms are prone to flabbiness as the years advance, and especially if you have had a dramatic weight loss through dieting.

So tone and firm up those muscles. This exercise is a particularly good one for generally strengthening the arms in preparation for many sports such as tennis, squash and ski-ing.

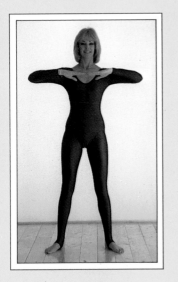

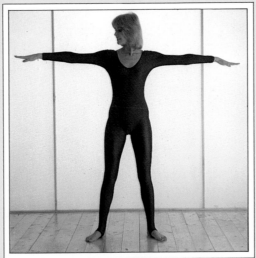

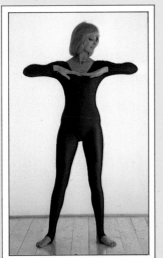

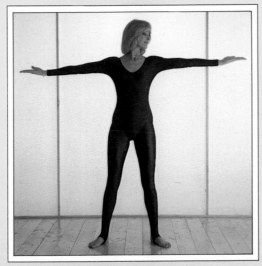

1 Stand or sit for this one. Raise arms up to shoulder level with the fingertips touching and palms down and elbows bent. Push back shoulders with two firm, strong movements

2 Open arms wide and fling back twice, working shoulders and expanding the chest

3 Bend elbows, fingertips touching again and push back twice

4 Fling open the arms, turning the palms upwards and push back twice. Then return to original position

● **REPEAT WHOLE MOVEMENT 6 TIMES** ●

Chest and Under Arms

Pull back your shoulders and improve your posture. This is an excellent exercise to expand the chest, release shoulder tension and tone up the under arms.

● **Do not attempt this exercise if you have any back problems.**

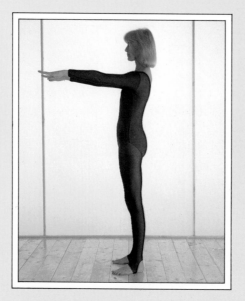

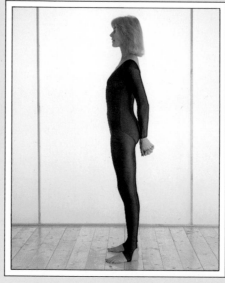

1 Stand with feet apart and arms out in front

2 Take the arms back behind your body, elbows straight and clasp hands together

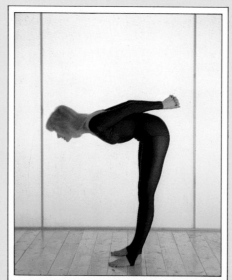

3 Pull in the tummy, bending over from the waist

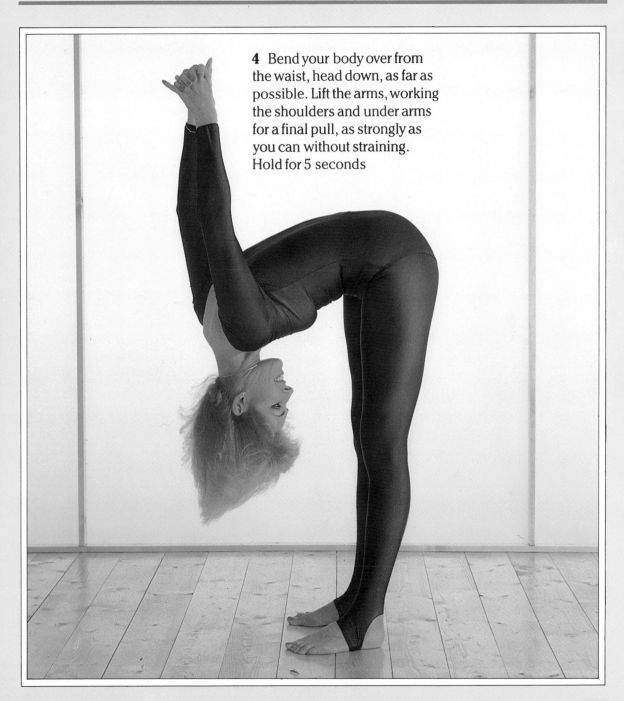

4 Bend your body over from the waist, head down, as far as possible. Lift the arms, working the shoulders and under arms for a final pull, as strongly as you can without straining. Hold for 5 seconds

Waist

Now you can whittle away your waist with this sideways stretch which will slim and trim the midriff.

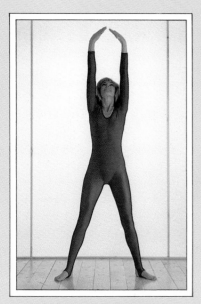

1 Stand with feet apart, arms stretched high above head, lifting up the rib cage

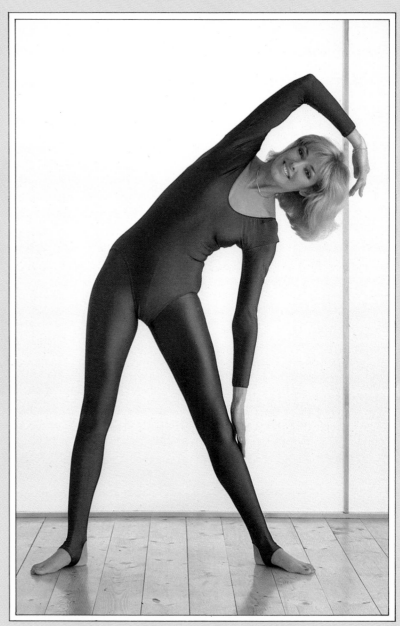

2 Bend the right arm over the head, pulling up and over and at the same time slide the left arm down the left leg bending over sideways from the waist only – keeping the hips steady. Give two little pushes down

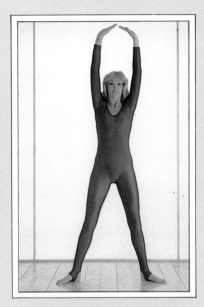

3 Straighten up and stretch both arms up high

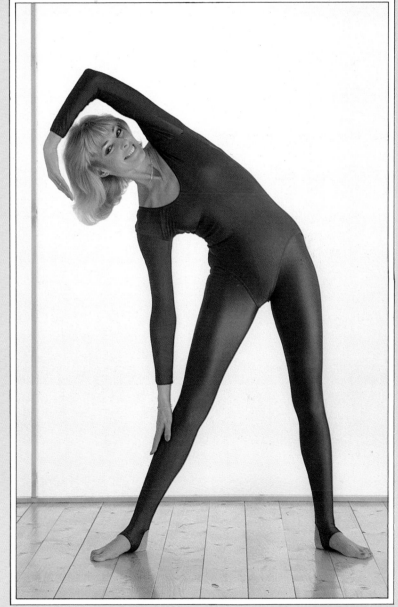

4 Curve the left arm up over the head, bending sideways from the waist and sliding the right arm down the right side. Push down twice – don't lean forward

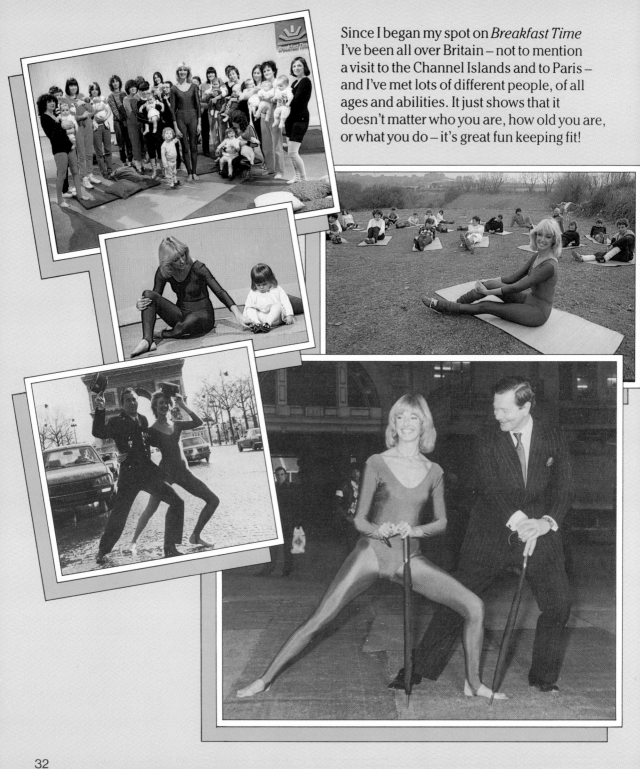

Since I began my spot on *Breakfast Time* I've been all over Britain – not to mention a visit to the Channel Islands and to Paris – and I've met lots of different people, of all ages and abilities. It just shows that it doesn't matter who you are, how old you are, or what you do – it's great fun keeping fit!

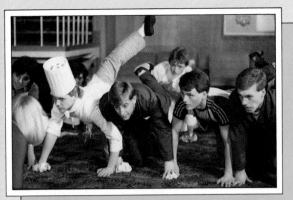

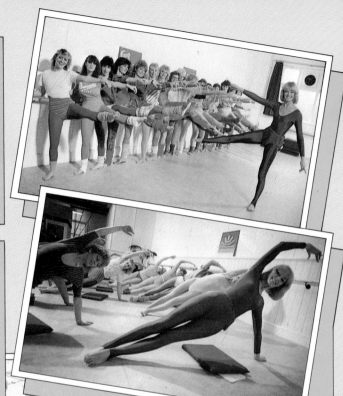

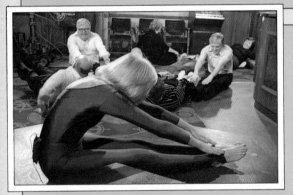

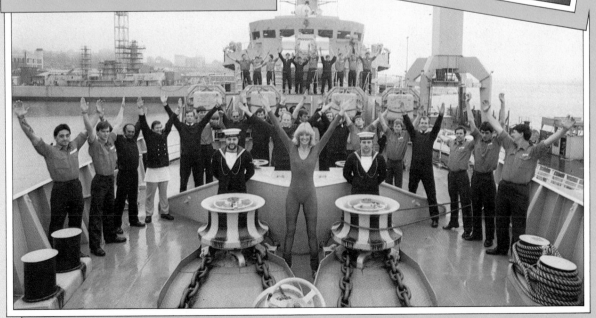

Waist and Back

Keep the back supple and mobile with this movement whilst you concentrate on your middle.

● **Don't forget — any exercise session must begin with a warm-up.**

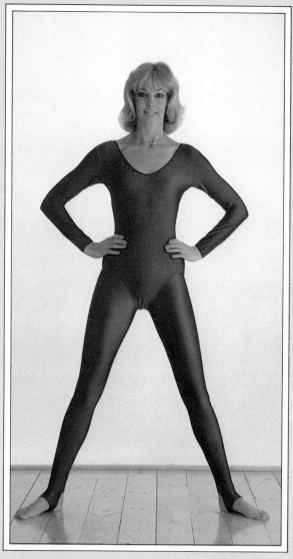

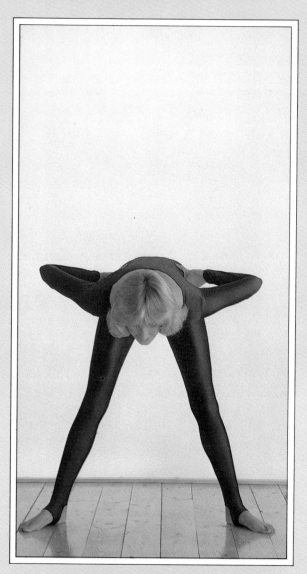

1 Stand with legs apart and hands on hips

2 Bend forward from the waist only

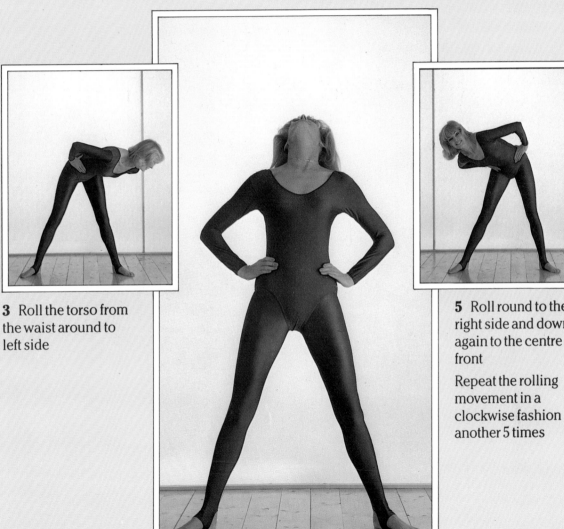

3 Roll the torso from the waist around to left side

4 Continue on around in a circular movement bending back

5 Roll round to the right side and down again to the centre front

Repeat the rolling movement in a clockwise fashion another 5 times

Tummy

The bulk of my problem letters come from people complaining about their tums. From men who have developed a beer gut, and many from ladies who have had babies and find it difficult to regain their figures. Also letters from both men and women who are showing signs of 'middle age spread'.

Don't think these problems are inevitable – they're not!
But, what they do need is plenty of willpower to improve them.
So now let's begin our 'Battle of the Bulge'.

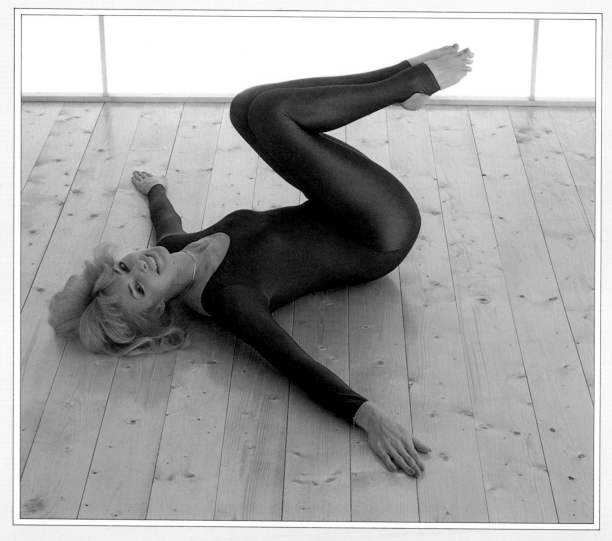

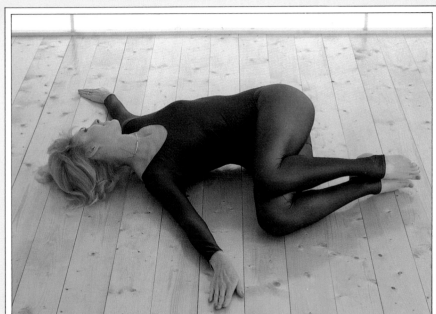

1 Lie on your back with your arms wide apart and pull up the knees to the chest

2 Twisting only from the waist, roll over to the left side, placing the bent knees to the floor. Keep your shoulders in contact with the floor

3 Pull up the knees and take them back to the centre and then roll on to the right

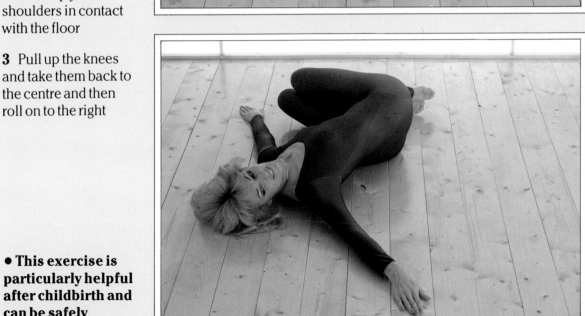

• **This exercise is particularly helpful after childbirth and can be safely started after your post-natal check**

Tummy and Thighs

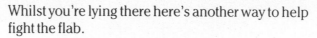

Whilst you're lying there here's another way to help fight the flab.

1 Lie flat on your back with your arms wide apart. Bend the knees to chest, then straighten up, pointing toes. Hold, then bring knees back to chest

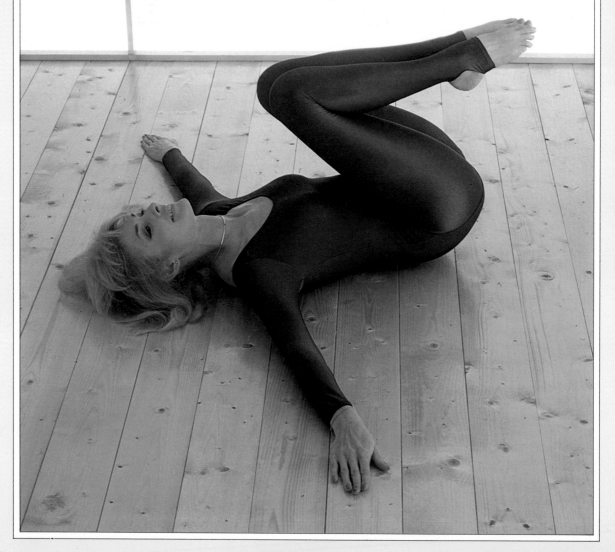

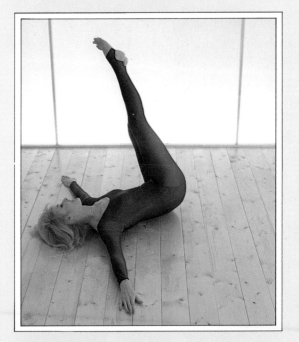

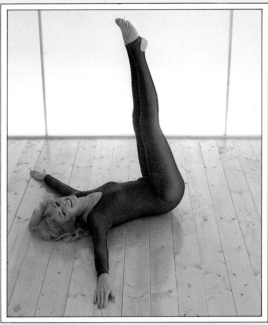

2 Twist from the waist to the left, straighten legs up and hold

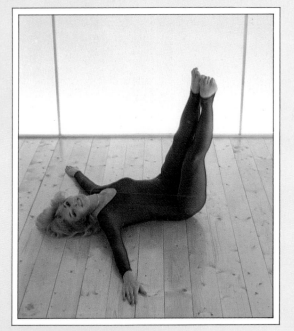

3 Return knees to chest and come back to the centre. Straighten legs up and hold

4 Twist from the waist to the right. Straighten legs up and hold, all the time keeping your shoulders in contact with the floor

Tummy and Hips

This is another simple exercise to help flatten the tum and it will keep the hips mobile too.

1 Lie on your back with your arms wide apart. Bend your right knee to the chest and then straighten the leg up

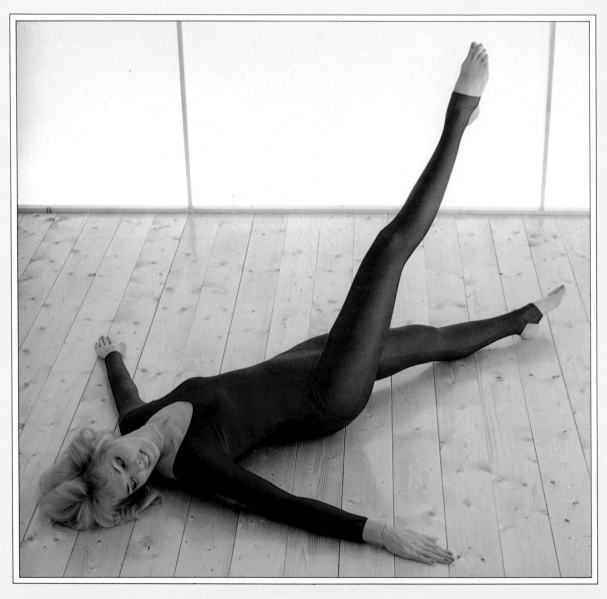

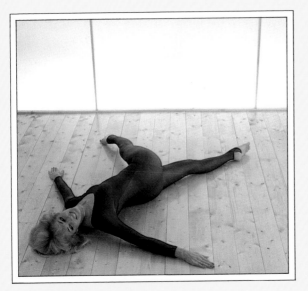

2 Keeping the shoulders firmly on the floor, take the straight leg over to the left side and touch the floor as near to your left hand as possible

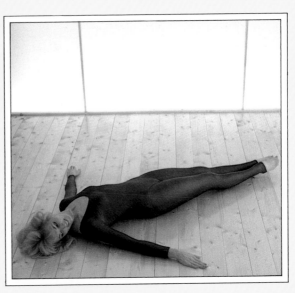

3 Bring leg back to centre and down to floor

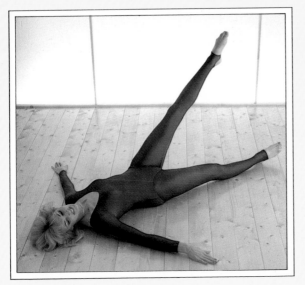

4 Lift the left leg and straighten it up

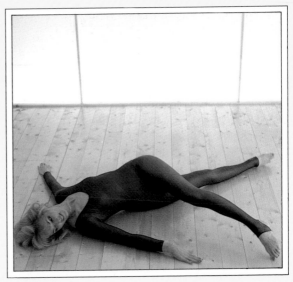

5 Touch the floor on the right side with the left leg

41

Middle

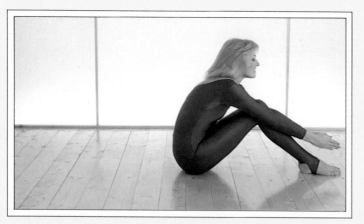

A classic pull-up now to help that tummy – gentle and effective – it helps keep the spine flexible too. A bed or a heavy piece of furniture can be a useful 'prop' at the start to hold down the feet until your muscles get stronger.

1 Sit with knees bent and feet flat on the floor. Curl forward over the knees with bent back. Raise the arms up by the side of the knees, hands pointing straight out to the front

2 Very slowly let the body go backwards. Keep the spine curled and the head up

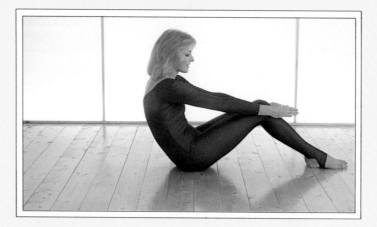

3 Gradually unroll the back and go down to the floor, vertebra by vertebra. Use the central tummy muscles and clench the buttocks to control and maintain the curled-up position

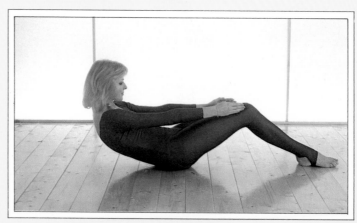

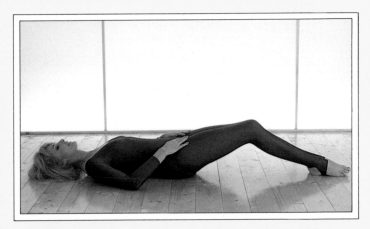

4 At the same time, slide the arms past the knees and onto the thighs. Go down flat and rest

5 Pull up slowly, raising the head and shoulders, hands by your knees and keeping spine curled over. Roll on up

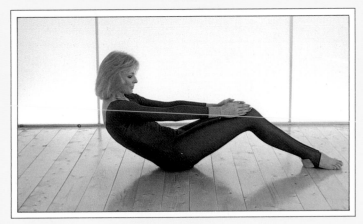

6 Back to the starting position. Relax!

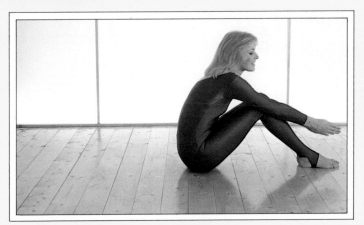

Hips

An exercise to keep the hips loose and the legs in great shape too! Feel those lazy inside thigh muscles!

The back of a chair or the bannister makes an ideal Barre – so improvise, there's no need to go to a gym. Even a member of your family or a friend could be used as support – it might encourage *them* to exercise!

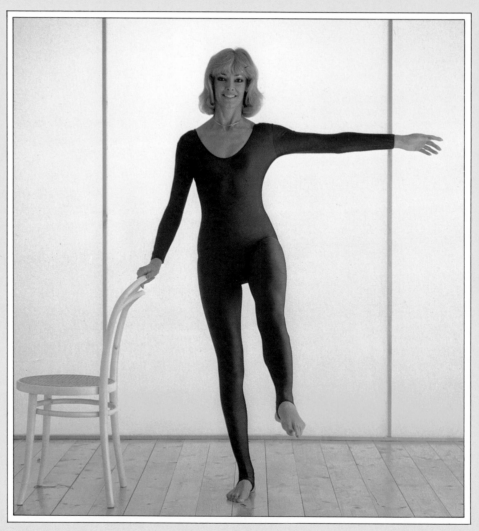

1 Hold on to the support with right arm, put the left arm out (like a ballet dancer) for balance

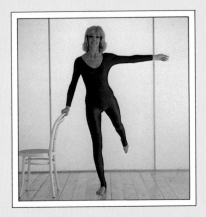

2 Continue by swinging the leg back

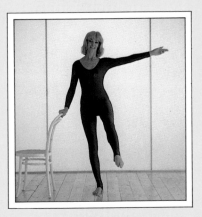

3 Swing to front again

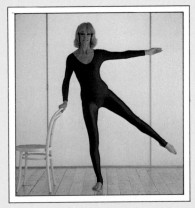

4 Keep the leg high, take it round to the left side

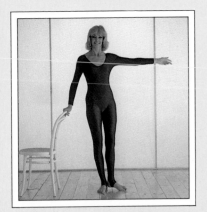

5 Drop it down to the floor

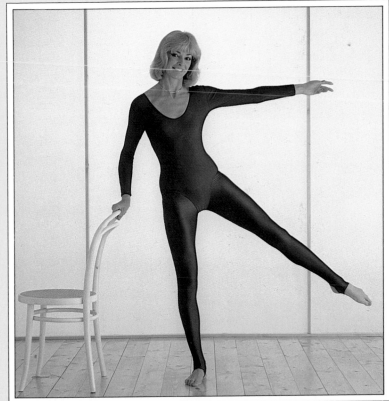

6 Quickly kick it up high again, then return to the ground

Bottom and Thighs

My mailbag could be equally divided between the two most common problem areas – tums and bums! Let's get to the bottom of it!

● **Do not attempt this exercise if you have any back problems**.

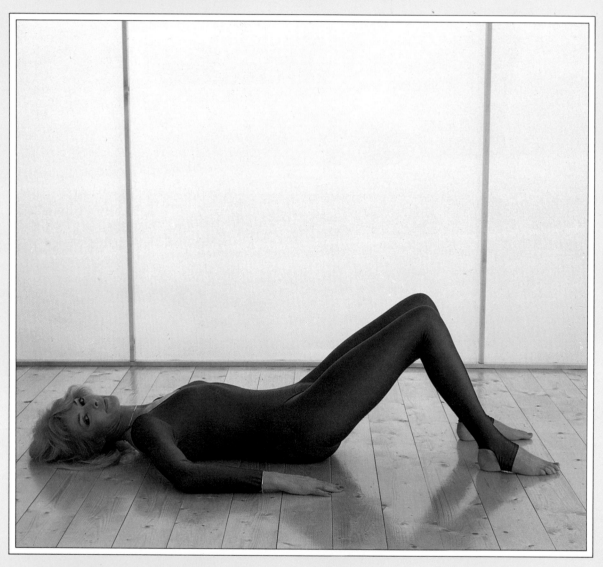

1 Lie on your back with arms at your sides. Knees bent and feet shoulder width apart and flat on the floor. Come down and relax

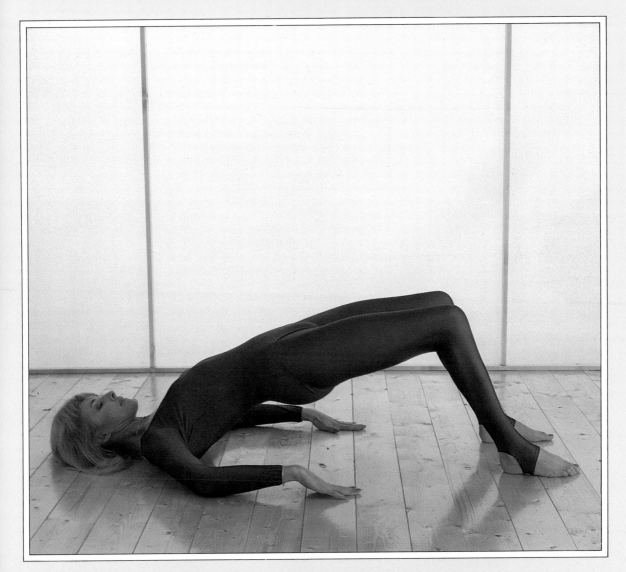

2 Clench the buttocks, pull in the tummy and lift the pelvis up high, transferring weight on to the shoulders. Hold for 5 seconds

Bottom and Legs

Don't just lie there – do something about it!

● **Do not attempt this exercise if you have a history of back trouble**.

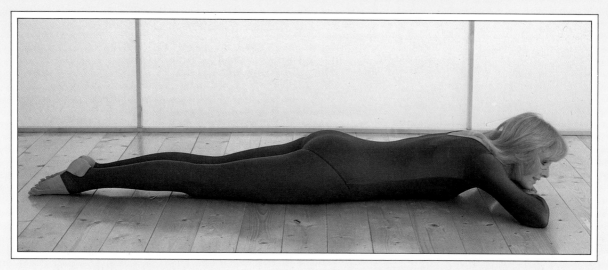

1 Lie on your tummy with your arms supporting your body at shoulder level and palms flat on the floor

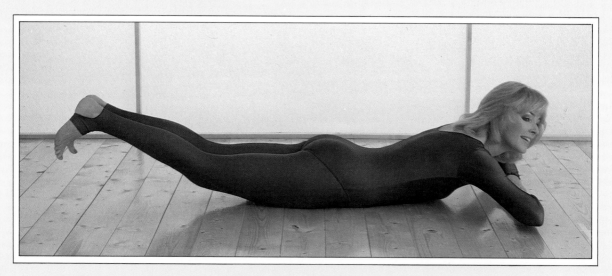

2 Press your pelvis into the floor and lift legs, feet together, toes pointed down. At the same time curve spine and lift head and shoulders

3 Kick legs out wide, turning the knee so that the toes are out and down

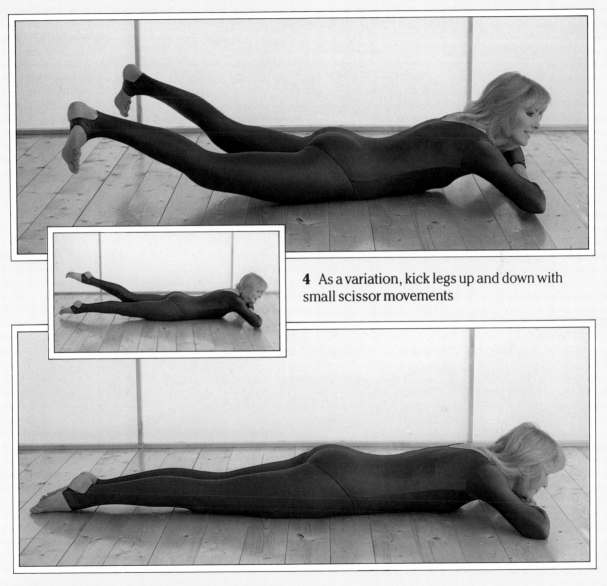

4 As a variation, kick legs up and down with small scissor movements

5 Return to original position and rest

Thighs

English ladies tend, on average, to be heavier on the thighs than their Latin cousins. Many are proportionally smaller in the bust resulting in the traditional 'pear shape'.

If heavy thighs are your problem, try this exercise for trimming and slimming the inner and outer thigh.

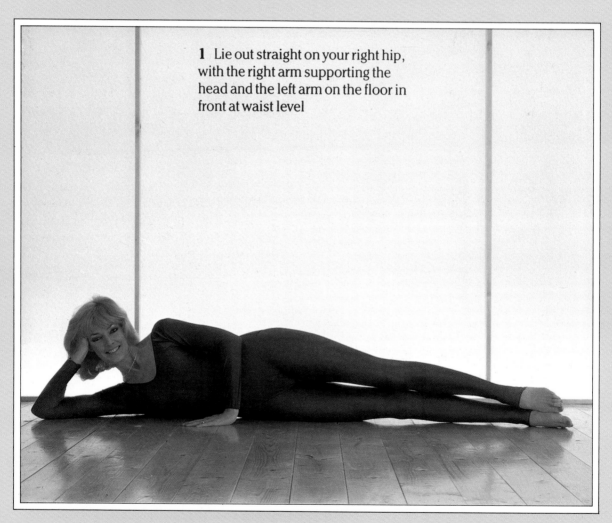

1 Lie out straight on your right hip, with the right arm supporting the head and the left arm on the floor in front at waist level

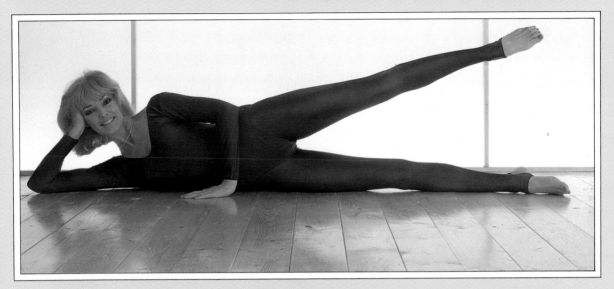

2 Raise up the top leg, pointing the toes. Keep the back straight and don't fall back or roll forward on the hip

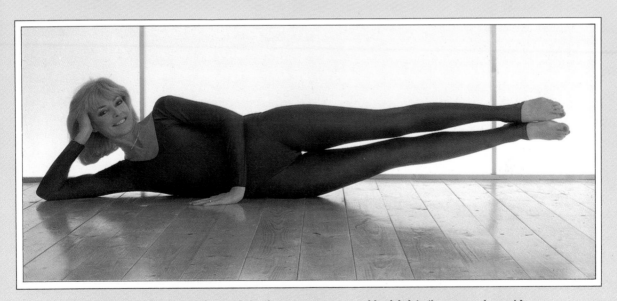

3 Bring up the lower leg to join the upper one and hold this 'banana shape' for 6 seconds. Keep thighs, calves and ankles together. Roll over and exercise the other side

Knees

Let's concentrate on the legs, keeping the hip, knee and ankle joints supple – strengthening and toning the thighs and calves.

● **Don't forget that before starting any sort of exercises you should have a thorough warm-up. This exercise is not recommended for anyone with a history of knee problems.**

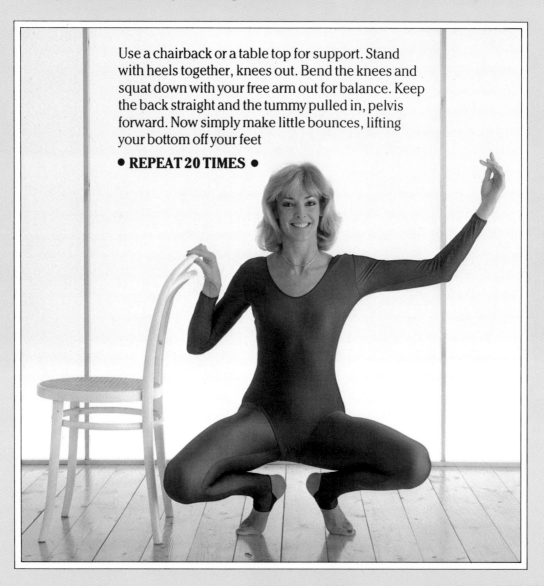

Use a chairback or a table top for support. Stand with heels together, knees out. Bend the knees and squat down with your free arm out for balance. Keep the back straight and the tummy pulled in, pelvis forward. Now simply make little bounces, lifting your bottom off your feet

● **REPEAT 20 TIMES** ●

Let's strengthen and shape up the legs and trim the seat too.

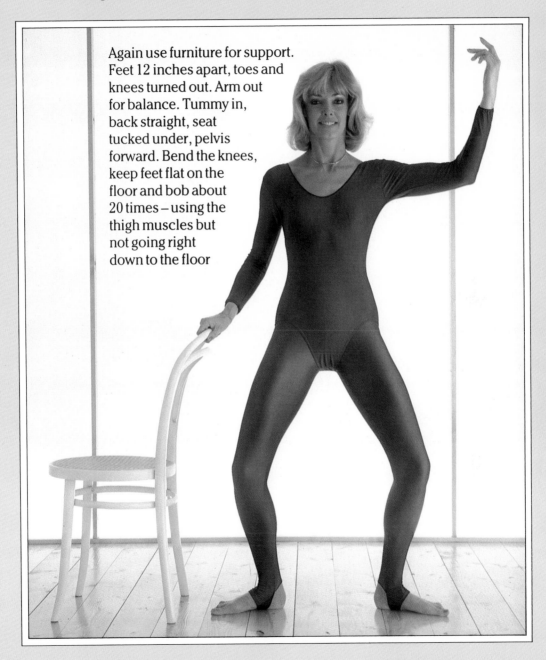

Again use furniture for support.
Feet 12 inches apart, toes and
knees turned out. Arm out
for balance. Tummy in,
back straight, seat
tucked under, pelvis
forward. Bend the knees,
keep feet flat on the
floor and bob about
20 times – using the
thigh muscles but
not going right
down to the floor

Calves

Don't neglect the muscles in the back of the legs which can shorten, particularly with constant wearing of high-heeled shoes. Try to stretch them gently.

● **Don't attempt this exercise or the next one if you have any problems with your back**

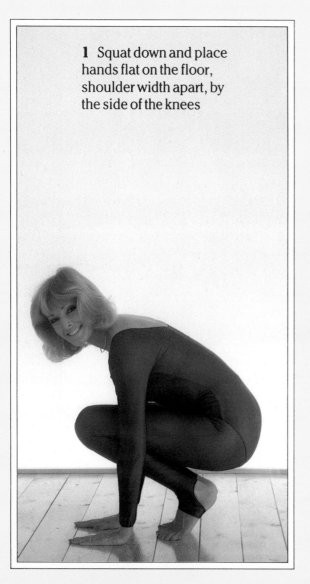

1 Squat down and place hands flat on the floor, shoulder width apart, by the side of the knees

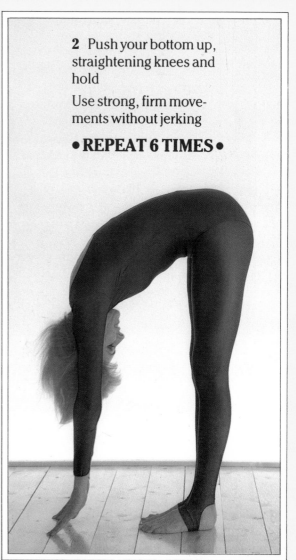

2 Push your bottom up, straightening knees and hold

Use strong, firm movements without jerking

●**REPEAT 6 TIMES**●

Spine

This is to stretch the back leg muscles and keep the spine supple.

1 Stand with the feet together, hands resting on thighs

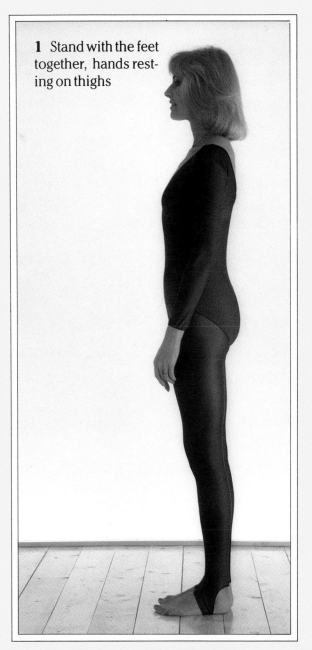

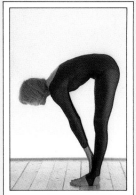

2 Pull in the tummy, drop head to chest and slowly bend the spine forward and over from the waist, sliding hands down over knees to ankles

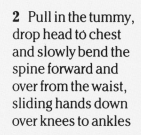

3 Take the hands to the back of the ankles and clasp them together

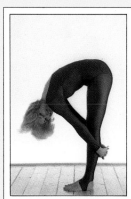

4 Bend elbows out and give an extra pull on hands bringing head to knee, or as far as you can comfortably go without straining. Hold for 6 seconds. Unclasp hands and slowly straighten up, uncurling the spine vertebra by vertebra to the upright position. This gets easier with practice and as the back leg muscles loosen

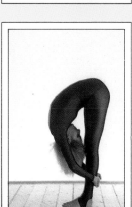

● **REPEAT 6 TIMES** ●

Ankles

Don't forget the ankles – for a pretty ankle can still turn plenty of heads. Strengthen and keep them trim with this simple routine.

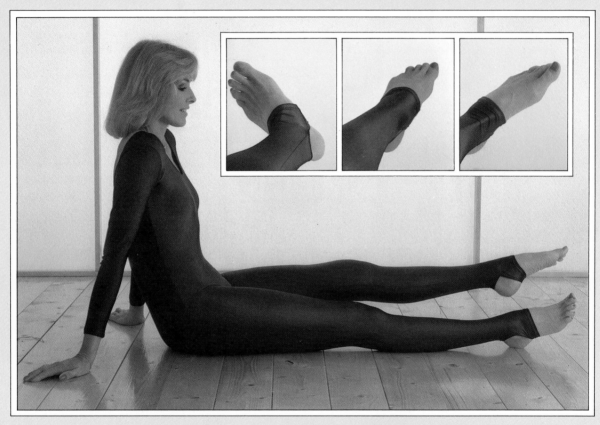

Sit down with legs straight out in front, hands on floor near your bottom for support. Sit up tall with a straight back and your tummy pulled in. Lift your left leg, then moving only the foot and ankle (not the entire leg), slowly and firmly make circles in a clockwise direction. Put leg down and rest. Raise right leg and repeat circling

Repeat, but moving feet in an anti-clockwise direction

• CIRCLE EACH FOOT 5 TIMES CLOCKWISE AND 5 TIMES ANTI-CLOCKWISE •

Feet

And finally the poor old feet! They're the only pair you have and they've a lot to put up with. Ill-treat them and they'll hurt and it'll show – in your face! So keep the feet supple and put a spring in your step, avoid that ageing shuffle with this simple stretch.

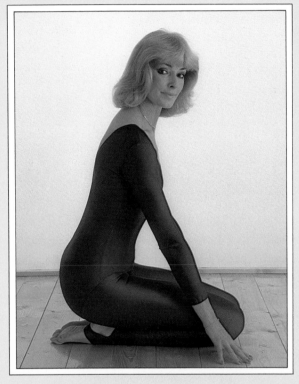

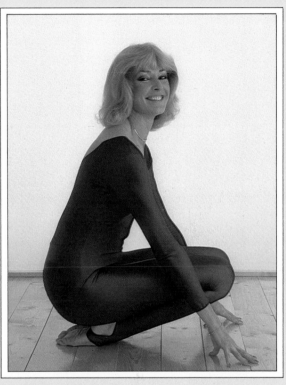

1 Kneel, bottom on feet, and place fingertips on floor by side of knees. Keep back straight and tummy in

2 Keep bottom on feet and lift up the knees only, stretching the front of the foot and ankles. Hold for 5 seconds, then bring knees down and rest

● **REPEAT 5 TIMES** ●

This hurts to begin with but gets easier with practice as the foot becomes more supple

Pass Out

But now you deserve a rest! So lie back and refresh the whole of your body.

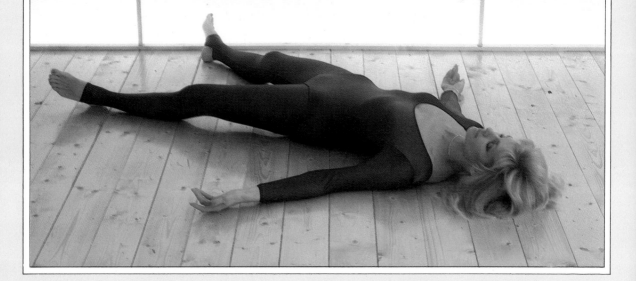

Lie on your back – legs out but relaxed. Let your knees and ankles flop out. Your arms should rest loosely on the floor away from your body, palms uppermost. Shoulders flat (lift up and move the upper torso if necessary to lessen the arch in your spine). Try to push your waist flat to the floor. Neck and shoulders relaxed – chin up. Breathe slowly and deeply. Fill and expand your lungs slowly, using the chest like bellows. Close your eyes and lie there for a few minutes and just *relax*

This is the end of the complete top-to-toe fitness routine.
On pages 59-64 are variations on some of the exercises which you might like to try...

Tummy and Thighs

A simple exercise as an alternative way to tone up the tummy muscles.

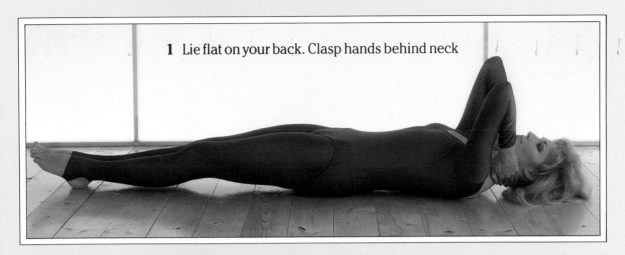

1 Lie flat on your back. Clasp hands behind neck

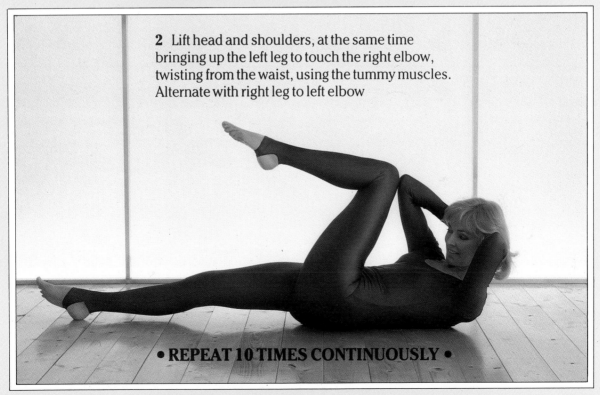

2 Lift head and shoulders, at the same time bringing up the left leg to touch the right elbow, twisting from the waist, using the tummy muscles. Alternate with right leg to left elbow

• **REPEAT 10 TIMES CONTINUOUSLY** •

Tummy and Legs

A simple exercise you can do while sitting on your chair.

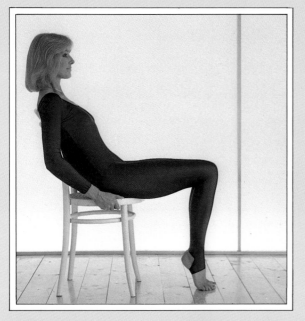

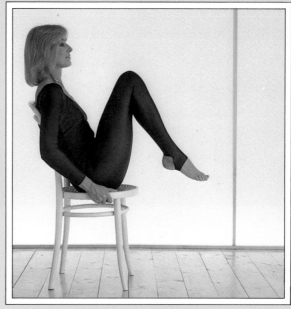

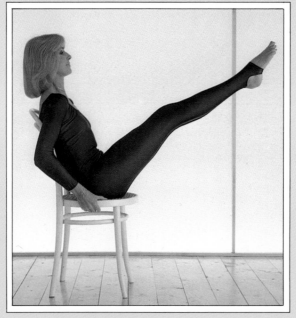

1 Slide your bottom forward so that the base of your spine is supported at the front of your chair, your shoulders well-supported by the back of the chair. Grasp the front of the chair firmly

2 Pull in the tummy bend the knees, and bring them up to the chest

3 Kick out and extend the legs. Hold for 5 seconds

• REPEAT 5 TIMES •

General Stretch

Feel a good stretch throughout the body and strengthen your back.

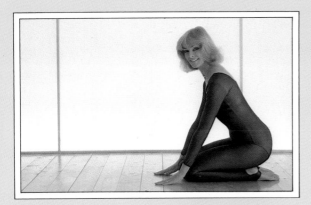

1 Kneel down, hands on the floor in front of knees

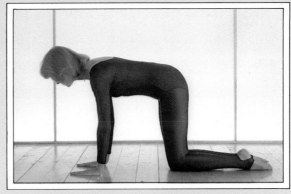

2 Slide hands forward and move body until you're on all fours with hands under shoulders

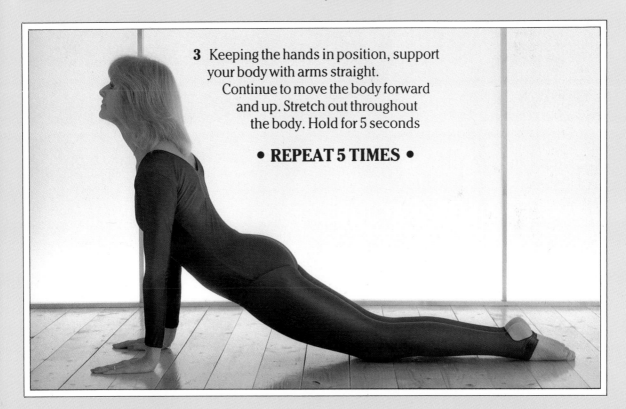

3 Keeping the hands in position, support your body with arms straight. Continue to move the body forward and up. Stretch out throughout the body. Hold for 5 seconds

• **REPEAT 5 TIMES** •

General Mobility

A nice way to keep the spine supple, the waist trim, and the arms and legs toned up.

● **Do not attempt this exercise if you have any back problems.**

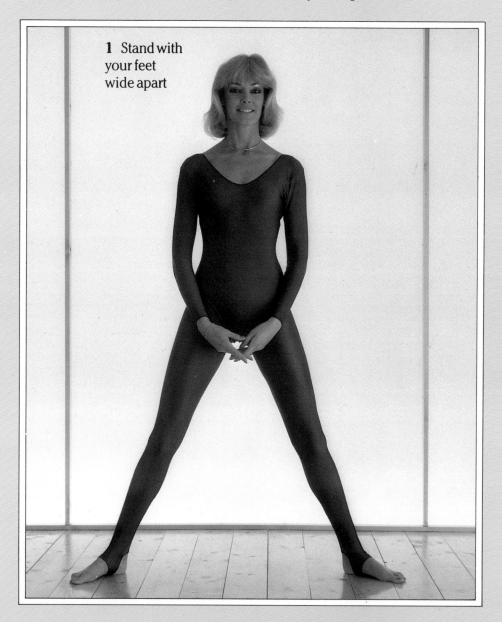

1 Stand with your feet wide apart

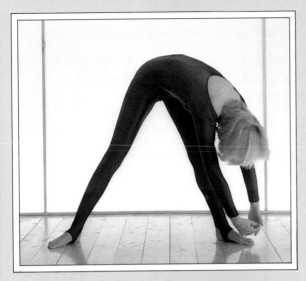

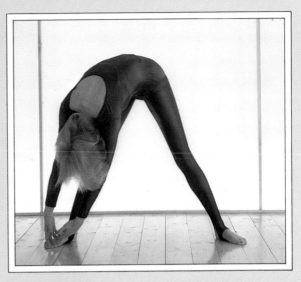

2 Bend over from the waist and make 2 little bounces with your hands touching your left foot or as near as possible

3 Swing the body up and over using your tummy muscles. Make 2 little bounces to the right foot. Over as far as you can go

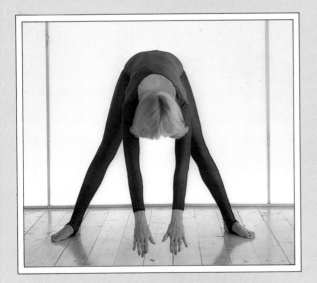

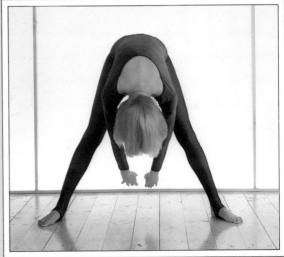

4 Swing up and reach forward as far as you can, your fingers touching the floor in front, with 2 little bounces

5 Then back through your legs and try to touch the floor behind as far as you can with 2 little bounces without straining

My Personal Pick-Me-Up

This is my salvation after a long day. It takes the weight off my feet, supports my aching back, clears my head and relaxes my whole body.

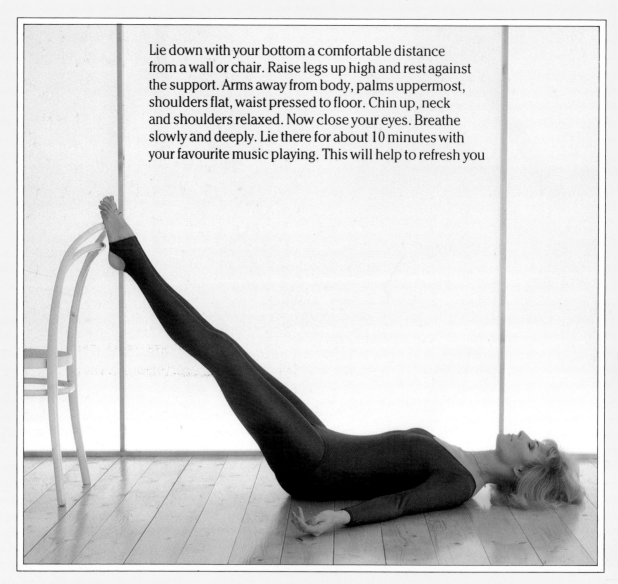

Lie down with your bottom a comfortable distance from a wall or chair. Raise legs up high and rest against the support. Arms away from body, palms uppermost, shoulders flat, waist pressed to floor. Chin up, neck and shoulders relaxed. Now close your eyes. Breathe slowly and deeply. Lie there for about 10 minutes with your favourite music playing. This will help to refresh you